Table of Contents

Understanding the Distinction Between Fear and Anxiety

1. Introduction to Fear and Anxiety

2. Historical Perspectives on Fear and Anxiety

3. Neurobiological Basis of Fear and Anxiety

Fear vs. Anxiety: Differences, Related Conditions, and More

1. Introduction

1.1. Purpose of the Work

1.2. Scope and Definition of Fear and Anxiety

2. Understanding Fear

There are two types of fear: primal and learned. Primal fear develops during childhood and is instinctual. Until roughly 3 years old, your child won't be afraid of the same things as adults because they haven't yet learned about them. More instincts as primal fears in adulthood can include fear of loud noises, falling, predators, and even social or separation from caregiver via illness or death. Learned fear is more prevalent in the tween and teenage years, but it's reasonable to experience for anyone. It happens when something isn't scary on its own, but then causes fear as a result of a traumatic experience, such as a car accident involving a loved one or a natural disaster. It becomes a phobia if the fear persists beyond this initial reaction, causing chronic or severe stress and interfering with daily life. Alongside adrenaline, noradrenaline, and other hormones, scientists also believe the amygdala (a part of the brain that helps process emotions) and preganglionic sympathetic neurons in the brain and spinal cord may be involved in the fear response. There appear to be noticeable differences between brain function when someone is a child and when the same person is an adult. Researchers are unsure how fear develops, but some possible factors include parenting style, anxiety in parents that passes to their kids, a genetic predisposition, and traumatic experiences. Drug and alcohol use has also been shown to impair the fear response system. Chronic or severe stress can also poison the brain and impair its functions, including fear and anxiety.

Fear is a normal emotional response to danger and is meant to protect you from harm. But when fear is irrational, excessive, and affects your daily life, it can be an indicator of anxiety. In the past, fear was considered a synonym of anxiety, but today the two terms are defined as distinct. Understanding fear is a fundamental step in getting to know what makes it different from anxiety.

2.1. Definition of Fear

Anxiety is a combination of a right response to alerting and resolving a possible scary scenario and also an improper psychological reaction to an outbreak that is difficult to safeguard. When fear goes unresolved to the spark that drives it, fear and anxiety will begin to assign to routine cases that, in fact, they do not warrant. When an individual is, nonetheless, acclimatized to their fears or anxieties, it may not hold major negative implications. But, this setback culture perpetuates, especially when an individual responds autonomously to opportunities for growth that are offered to them.

Fear is a very normal, physiological, and emotional response to a realistic and current danger or imminent threat. This quick, defensive response is not actually characterized as anxiety. Though anxiety performs a similar biological function, it is provoked by an indistinct or long-term stressor, rather than a real threat or threat. Early isolation once may have revealed practical application as a means of safety from hazardous scenarios.

2.2. Types of Fear

As early as 1925, the American behaviorist John Watson pointed out that there are at least two types of fear: simple fears of things or situations (which are the focus of phobias) and social fear. According to researchers from the area of cognitive psychology, there are, in fact, at least six identifiable types of fears. First of all, there are of course the "actual fears" or "external fears" of specific objects or situations. Moreover, there are simple, and then there are complex, specific threats. Whereas simple threats pose a clear and present danger, so-called anticipatory threats signify that a dangerous situation may occur at some point in the future.

Before diving deeper into our discussion of anxiety and fear, it is important to gain a clearer understanding of what fear is—and fear, it turns out, is a multifaceted phenomenon. Specific fears, also termed "phobias," were famously categorized by the behavioral psychologist Joseph Wolpe along a single dimension—an approach which has been modified by subsequent scientists. However, whereas phobias are characterized by the fact that they are closely tied to specific situations and objects—flying, heights, spiders, or interacting with people, for example—they actually do not make up the entirety of what we call "fear." Indeed, fear can manifest in a number of different ways.

2.3. Causes of Fear

Hormones. Hormonal disorders can cause many of the exhaustion symptoms. Diabrosis, overactive thyroid, adrenal cancer, and other hormonal changes may all cause anxiety.

Trauma or personal harm. Several situations may generate a fear response. Moreover, more people might experience fear later in life when things happen or what inevitably makes them feel insecure. When people are or have been mistreated, bodily violated, or yelling, several of them are afraid of being insulted. We may be harmed or humiliated and thus avoid the assault as a result. A past happening of physical, sexual, sexual, or emotional hurt could predict the future. Finally, it is common for people to suffer from PTSD after natural disasters, injuries, or illnesses. Almost 77% of people experience intense and lasting disease of at the very least 6 months before searching for medication. Rehabilitation of natural disaster visits patients, the patient Emergency Room, gets a drug, and regular nursing but never gets professional rehabilitation.

Personality. This could sound that when we overhear a cacophobic reaction – the fear of things that aren't well – personality might be the cause.

A feeling of fear over money. The money problem is a major cause of fear. The usual response to financial hardship is to be cautious and avoid falling freely into anxiety.

Everything that happens now, has been ended in the past, or is expected to happen in the future may be terrifying. Fear could potentially endanger a person. Understanding the various causes and forms of terror is important for selecting care for it. I think that there are several possible sources of fear. Here are a few factors to consider:

People usually become frightened or expect a terrible event whenever they anticipate fear. Some people develop it just by hearing about someone else's experience with it or because of something legal or historical. Several factors can influence fear, tension, and anxiety. Anxiety, worry, and tension have a significant influence on tension and anxiety.

3. Understanding Anxiety

If there are several sorts of anxiety, are there any shared risk factors that are common to all of them or more likely to occur in at least one subtype of anxiety disorder than not? There are a few clear highlights in the literature regarding increased likelihood for one or more anxiety disorders and these vulnerability factors: phenotypic anxiety (worry and fear), exposure to acute or chronic stress and trauma, and fear-generalization. It is not surprising that the degree to which these factors occur would matter. Misfortune, acute stress, and trauma can result in more symptomatology. Some people under stress will show anxiety up to a point (stress vulnerability factors), and some will not. There has been some support in the literature about the fact that this general lack of preference to show anxiety may also have some genetic influences. More work is needed in this domain, as are comparisons of samples using similar experiments to warrant that conclusions are sound.

Anxiety is a state of worry or unease, but not all states of unease are anxiety. For example, fear is a response to immediate threats, whereas anxiety occurs in reaction to situations perceived as a looming challenge or danger. Unlike fear, which disappears after a threat is resolved, anxiety can be a pervasive feeling of dread that endures for months or years. Distinct from the fear of an immediate threat or danger, anxiety exists in response to the anticipation of a perceived threat that may potentially come to pass at an indeterminate time in the future. Anxiety is a mood state that can range from worry to severe states where thoughts are out of control and it is very difficult to focus on tasks. People who express high levels of anxiety could also be diagnosed with an anxiety disorder. There are several types of anxiety disorders. These include generalized anxiety, panic disorder, social anxiety, and separation anxiety.

3.1. Definition of Anxiety

Much like fear, anxiety can cause physical and mental symptoms that may result in panic and other disorders. Anxiety is just the result of living life while fear is the result of specific or immediate predecessors. The definition seems even more fuzzy when we apply the term to medical conditions. In fact, it seems that as we apply the term progressively to tools, medications, therapies, and even to marketing strategies, that its meaning becomes less and less clear. Terms such as performance anxiety, separation anxiety, and anxiety of influence capture the idea that anxiety exists as an acute or chronic condition (with or without identifiable source of the fear), appears as a symptom of early or late-stage mental illness, and also might appear in an otherwise healthy, tension-ridden person. As a bad feeling or an ominous sign of worse to come, it may appear much like fear but exist just under the conscious surface making it more difficult for an individual to use cognitive work to alter.

The official definition of anxiety is "a feeling of worry, nervousness, or unease, typically about an imminent event or something with an uncertain outcome." It's a natural part of life that almost everyone will experience from time to time. It's known to protect you from physical danger by triggering your "fight-or-flight" response. But if you're not in physical danger, persistent feelings of worry can be overwhelming and disabling. In a 2004 article published in Occupational Medicine, a majority of workers surveyed reported feeling moderate or extremely stressed about work. This amounted to an upward of $300 billion of lost time and workplace productivity.

There are several different categories of anxiety, though a person experiencing any type of anxiety may also struggle with symptoms from other categories or symptoms of additional fearful conditions. There are also other anxiety-like and associated conditions that are considered debilitating or phobic.

- Generalized Anxiety: Generalized anxiety is what most people think of when they think of anxiety. It's what the DSM-5 manual refers to as general anxiety disorder (GAD) and is characterized by persistent, severe anxiety that goes past what is "normal" in a given situation. Generalized anxiety can present as exaggerated fears and worries more days than not for at least six months. Physical symptoms may include feeling wound up or on edge, being easily fatigued, difficulty concentrating or mind going blank, irritability, muscle tension, and sleep problems. - Panic Attacks/Panic Disorder: Panic attacks are sudden occurrences of intense fear and severe physical symptoms even though there is no real danger present. A panic attack reaches a peak within minutes, can happen in a variety of situations and sometimes unexpectedly. Symptoms can include a rapid or pounding heartbeat, trembling or shaking, shortness of breath or a "smothering" feeling, and feelings of choking. A person having a panic attack may feel dizzy, unsteady, lightheaded, or faint. They may also feel detached from themselves or reality.

It's important to note that a person with one type of anxiety can also experience another type, additional mental health conditions, or both. These can show up in different ways according to environmental, physical, mental, and situational factors.

3.3. Causes of Anxiety

Fear can be defined as the response to danger and the canonical scenario of not knowing about the anxiety triggers when danger is not present or necessarily tied to triggers. Nevertheless, research on fear helps to understand some of the phenomenon that anxiety presents. At least some aspects seen in people with anxiety disorder (as well as normal people) are shared across the rodent species in experimental paradigms that can study anxiety or its opposite, safety. Anxiety alone emanates from a mix of genetic, infectious, physical trauma, emotional trauma, life-course, and therapy factors. Neurobiological and some social factors have conserved cross-species mechanisms. There is currently no explanation for all these causes or for which piece is the most important. In addition, there appears to be familial sharing among these factors. Both normal and clinical (abnormal intensity and low quality of life) anxiety are present across different ages and in offspring to likely similar degree.

The possibility of causes is a side of anxiety that brings perspective. Just as anxiety is made of physiological systems, it is made of a variety of systems that could possibly go awry. It can come with a disability label, meaning that anxiety for some individuals comes with another mental or physical explanation; for others, this may not be the case and the anxiety remains unexplained or topographical. Anxiety worries and agitates both without and in the presence of fear responses.

Breadth of Anxiety

4. Differences Between Fear and Anxiety

Someone feeling fear might experience symptoms and exhibit behaviors such as trembling, sweating, rapid heartbeat, dry mouth, and an urge to flee. In comparison, someone suffering from anxiety may experience a more general list of symptoms and exhibit behaviors such as muscle tension, restlessness, physical fatigue, concentration difficulties, irritability, and difficulty with sleep. Physiologically, anxiety activates the body's threat response system. Still, it is predominantly experienced in the upper chest. Anxiety activates the survival mechanisms, triggering the well-known "fight or flight" response. Fear, on the other hand, is processed by the amygdala in the human brain. The amygdala allows us to react more quickly to the emotional content while processing information. In turn, this quick processing leads to hyperarousal, likely within the body's threat response system. Both of these factors create the emotional and behavioral experiences associated with phobias.

Fear and anxiety often accompany similar situations and cause similar symptoms, but they are distinct emotional states that are related to varying conditions and treated differently. Fear is emotionally charged but more specifically rooted in a clear and present threat, while anxiety tends to occur in confrontation with a more uncertain or general threat. In comparison, fear is a response to a known threat, and anxiety is a response to an unknown threat.

4.1. Key Characteristics

The fear sets off the battle-flight-freeze stress response and activates various parts of the brain that help you prepare for an instantaneous physical reaction. For example, to respond to the threat and help you flee, your pulse and heartbeat quicken. Fear is your immediate, emotional response to an identified or recognizable core. It moves on its own and is often tied to anything particular. Before and after you talk in front of a big crowd, you may not feel worried, but you may fear the specific situation. Fear isn't the safest feeling in the world, but it definitely serves a particular purpose. Anxiety, on the other hand, is distinguished by its ambiguity. There is no realistic or observable source of risk associated with anxiety. Yes, it is frequently the product of thinking about the future, and this future may include anything frightening.

Fear and anxiety are both intense emotional states that are frequently linked and frequently mistaken for one another. One of the most significant differences between the two is that fear arises in the presence of a challenging situation, such as when you are hiking and are abruptly face to face with a snarling bear.

In some ways, anxiety can be thought of as an inappropriate activating of the "fight or flight" response. In response to a "perceived threat," the amygdala stimulates a number of brain regions, the hypothalamus, which activates the autonomic nervous system through the sympathetic nervous system. Like fear, anxiety can be associated with physiological "fight or flight" reactions. However, these symptoms may occur even when there is no actual threat to motivate them. This is why some people find it hard to think of anxiety as a form of fear. Furthermore, whereas fear is an emotional reaction to an actual threat, anxiety is an emotional reaction to a subjective judgment of a potential threat.

When facing a threatening situation, the amygdala, a key part of the limbic system, is activated. The amygdala processes the sensory data and sends input to different parts of the brain. The projections to the hypothalamus cause the characteristic features of the "fight or flight" response. The hypothalamus activates the autonomic nervous system by sending nerve signals through the sympathetic nervous system. The sureotips of the hypothalamus also stimulate the release of adrenaline from the adrenal medulla, enhancing the fight or flight response. There are several physiological changes associated with the activation of the fight or flight response, including increases in heart rate, blood pressure, and breathing rate.

4.3. Behavioral Responses

In addition to the responses to unconditioned and conditioned stimuli, there are also behavioral differences between fear and anxiety in conflict paradigms. The administration of D-cycloserine, a glycine-site partial NMDA agonist, has been found to facilitate the extinction of cued fear, whereas benzodiazepines do not. Research has confirmed that benzodiazepines treat state anxiety, whereas flumazenil can reverse the anti-anxiety effects of benzodiazepines in humans. Benzodiazepines are also known to specifically abate anxiety but not phobic responding. The negative affect that is missing in persons suffering from psychopathy is responsible for the avoidance response deficit, as well as the abnormal fear conditioning. In more recent research, the most reliable results regarding the behavioral differences were the following: avoidance behavior recovered earlier in cued fear than anxiety with fear conditioning, but humans who received anxiolytic treatment avoided sooner than controls in an avoidance conflict with mixed fear conditioning.

There are a variety of behavioral responses representing fear and anxiety, and the collection has suggested that there is not a one-to-one correspondence between any one behavioral response and either fear or anxiety. A review of the literature on behavioral responses to cued and contextually conditioned fear and anxiety will demonstrate that interference with operant responding can suppress anxiety but not fear, while the presentation of a discriminative stimulus that allows subjects to avoid an aversive event will suppress fear but not anxiety.

5. Similarities Between Fear and Anxiety

It can be difficult to know exactly what someone is experiencing just by looking at them or listening to how they describe their feelings. That said, there are quite a few similarities between fear and anxiety. Some symptoms of fear cause physical sensations, such as a racing heart or fast breathing. Anxiety can cause physical symptoms, too, like muscle tension and increased heart rate, but it rarely comes on as quickly as fear. While someone experiencing fear may experience a feeling of imminent danger, anxiety can sometimes feel like a much more general fear. As far as phobias go, fear and phobias can be experienced even when the feared object or situation is not present. Someone with social anxiety, for instance, may spend all day worrying about what will happen at a party planned for the evening. Anxiety makes the world look threatening in a general way rather than evoking fear about a particular thing or event. Fears tend to pop up and seem momentarily intractable.

Fear and anxiety are unpleasant emotional states that cause mental, physical, and behavioral changes. Fear is usually a reaction to a specific danger. For example, if someone is home alone and hears a loud, unexplained noise, they might feel fear. But anxiety can occur without a life-threatening situation, and it doesn't always disappear when the situation resolves. Anxiety is also more difficult to manage and can last for long periods of time. At its onset, anxiety can feel vague and unsettling, but symptoms can escalate quickly. Because they have different triggers and durations, it's important to address the two emotions differently to manage them more effectively. Treating anxiety involves learning more about how it occurs and when it's at its worst. It involves retraining the brain and the body to behave differently than it has been used to.

5.1. Common Symptoms

In cognitive behavior, there will be thinking or feeling that they are being insulted or despised. On emotional and bodily levels, the same situation gives rise to anger or fear, with an increased heart rate and rapid breathing. The cognitive level is affected, or there is altered thinking by one's emotional status. The emotional aspects consist of uneasiness, tension, stress, depression, and strain. However, both sides of the pathological state also have their specific symptoms. So, in traditional teaching, on fear, the focus tends to be on the cognitive level, with little attention paid to the emotional level, while in anxiety, the "opposite" observation is probably made.

The common symptoms between fear and anxiety are the experience of physical, cognitive, and emotional arousal. The physiological symptoms or physical indicators consist of a rise in blood pressure and body temperature, quickened heartbeat, tightened muscles, shortness of breath, stomach cramps, colic, and diarrhea. Profusely sweating, cramps in grip muscles, frequent rigors, rush of adrenaline, vertigo, hot or cold flush, choking in the throat, confusion, and tension headache are also experienced by people in general suffering from fear and anxiety. A dry mouth, difficulty in swallowing, and an acidic feeling in the mouth are some of the other indicators experienced by many anxious people. The cognitive aspect consists of a loss of alertness or concentration, paranoia, or even panic. Although fear and anxiety have physiological symptoms, it is the mental status that is most affected.

Common Symptoms:

5.2. Impact on Daily Life

Similarly, a person experiencing fear can mask it at times, but there are moments and situations where the fear is visible. Their lives can revolve around this fear and completely change their lifestyle. These can lead to legal trouble if they cause physical harm to someone, loss of employment, or other strained relationships. There are irrational phobias, which can lead to a social loss depending on the specific fear, such as the fear of leaving one's home. For example, fear can become physical, leading to heart racing, sweating, and shaking, just as with anxiety. The difference is that with anxiety, it can happen within the safety of one's home or with a familiar group of people. Therefore, fear and anxiety can both alter normal daily living.

Having symptoms of anxiety and extreme anxiousness can lead to catastrophizing or overthinking potential situations. This can lead to questionable choices, self-medicating through substance use or over-the-counter items, strained relationships, issues with employment, and at times legal troubles. Repetitive behaviors and activities such as handwashing, seeking constant reassurance, checking on loved ones to ensure that they are not hurt, etc., can lead to a high number of arguments with others who see these things as being taken to extremes.

6. Related Conditions

Just like fear and anxiety are not the same, these conditions and symptoms can overlap. Childhood and separation anxiety disorders, for example, are characterized by overwhelming, intense worry. In some people, anxiety can also appear as a symptom of phobias, panic disorder, and obsessive-compulsive disorder. Despite these connections, people can have fears, phobias, and related conditions without having anxiety.

3. Generalized Anxiety Disorder: While many people might worry about money, a relationship, or a recent natural disaster, some people have persistent, overwhelming worry that disrupts daily life. For example, a person with generalized anxiety disorder might be unable to focus on other tasks due to their constant worry, even if there's nothing they can do to address the situation immediately.

2. Panic Disorder: People with panic disorder experience episodes of intense fear, commonly known as panic attacks. Sometimes, panic attacks can occur without an obvious trigger. Though they usually don't pose much of a threat, some symptoms of a panic attack—like a rapid heart rate and chest pain—resemble symptoms of health conditions such as a heart attack.

1. Phobias: While it's common to feel scared of something, people who have phobias have intense fears of objects, activities, or situations. Sometimes, these fears can inhibit the ability to perform daily activities. For example, some

people might be so scared of snakes that they are unable to spend time outside.

Sometimes, fear and anxiety can develop into conditions that impact daily living. Here are a few closely related conditions to explore:

6.1. Phobias

The Diagnostic and Statistical Manual of Mental Disorders-5 (DSM-5) classifies a specific phobia (SP) as a marked fear or anxiety about a specific object or situation; for children, the parent may present the fear. Minimal exposure to the phobic stimulus can be the cause of the fear. People with SP may experience avoidance of seeing the phobic object (in the case of animal phobias), anticipation of a bad event when the phobic object appears (in the case of situational or environmental phobias), heart racing, shortness of breath, trembling and shaking, nausea or other gastrointestinal symptoms, poor comprehension, confusion, or dizziness. A past study conducted with 921 college students reported that the most commonly reported specific phobias among them were gephyrophobia (fear of crossing bridges), gynophobia (fear of women), and phobophobia (fear of having a phobia).

A phobia is one type of fear-related condition experienced by an individual. People with phobias have a significant, persistent fear of specific things or situations, even when they know that the fear is unreasonable. There are many specific phobias, including acarophobia (fear of insects that cause itching), ophidiophobia (fear of snakes), pediculophobia (fear of lice), and zemmiphobia (fear of the great mole rat); animals are the most common phobia stimuli. Phobia can occur due to an unpleasant initial experience, a series of experiences in which the stimuli are associated with pain or bad news, a direct experience of a fearful event, exposure to a fearful event, or being told of a terrible experience by others.

6.2. Panic Disorder

Individuals with panic disorder present with a rapid unprovoked onset of panic attacks, with the onset of them ranging from minutes to about 10 minutes, and they are highly prevalent in females. Types of panic disorder: There are two types of panic disorder, one with agoraphobia and one without. Agoraphobia is the fear or avoidance of places and situations that might cause fear and panic. The relationship between agoraphobia and panic disorder is controversial, and while it is certainly comorbid with panic disorder (about 55–75% of cases also have agoraphobia), it is actually quite rare to have agoraphobia without a diagnosis of panic disorder. In other words, it might well be that both conditions are two sides of the same coin; or alternatively, the disability associated with panic attacks might give rise to agoraphobia in the individual. Panic attacks can also occur infrequently in non-agoraphobic people, in which case they would not have a diagnosis of panic disorder. Panic disorder is associated with substantial comorbid psychopathology; those with it are likely to suffer from one or more present comorbid conditions alongside panic disorder. Panic disorder is also associated with a high level of suicidality. Panic disorder is generally treated biologically, with the use of antidepressants, benzodiazepines, or cognitive-behavioral therapy.

Panic disorder is a discrete subclass of anxiety-related condition. DSM-IV restricted the diagnosis of panic disorder to individuals of at least 18 years of age, and a diagnosis of panic disorder was not to be given if the onset of panic attacks was drug or substance use related or due to a general medical condition. The lifetime prevalence of panic disorder in adults ranges between 2.4% and 5.1%. Panic disorder has a high comorbidity with other psychiatric disorders, and panic attacks occur as part of the symptomatology of other conditions, from the affective disorders to the anxiety-related conditions; however, the presentation is different.

Discrete subclass of anxiety-related condition: Background and characteristics

It can be challenging to treat GAD. However, both medicinal and non-drug therapies have been seen to alleviate this disorder. If you think you or a loved one has GAD, you should consider speaking with a healthcare professional. Anxiety, on its own, is not a one-size-fits-all diagnosis. People experience and feel anxiety in different ways, and there are many different types of anxiety disorders that can be diagnosed. ADHD, obsessive-compulsive disorder (OCD), social phobias, or panic attacks are examples of these symptoms. One of the most common types of anxiety disorder seen in the general population is simple phobias. Nevertheless, the most common type of anxiety disorder seen in mental health facilities is generalized anxiety disorder (GAD). GAD is characterized by unpleasant thoughts or significant stress over issues like financial problems, health, or family. The panic and mood disorders are highly associated with GAD and with each other. People who have GAD often also have depression and panic disorders.

One of the most common mental health conditions in the United States is generalized anxiety disorder (GAD). Not only can it be debilitating physically and emotionally, but it can also make daily life difficult. GAD is a type of anxiety disorder that is characterized by constant and excessive stress over several months. If someone has GAD, they may feel as though there is nothing they can do to relieve anxiety. Some individuals with GAD worry excessively about daily life activities, such as money, family, work, or health.

7. Diagnosis and Treatment

7.1. Diagnostic Criteria

7.2. Assessment Tools

7.3. Therapeutic Approaches

8. Conclusion

Both anxiety and fear play a significant role in a comprehensive conceptualization of psychopathologies where emotional hyper-reactivity and increased sensitivity towards punishment are important. Nevari et al. designed an intervention which focuses on challenging safety behaviors, a common feature of both anxiety and fear (including phobias) which can maintain distress and the anxious/fearful cycle. Disputing safety behaviors and the post's emphasis on people getting through real-time feared scenarios is a way-led approach. Research also has a biological narrative to understand when fear and anxiety become problematic through the stress response system. "Initially, the sympathetic-adreno-medullary system reacts to stress primarily through the secretion of catecholamines by the adrenal medulla, before the activation of the endocrine system. This system helps to modulate vegetative functions and manage fear-related responses." It could be beneficial to explore some research around the role of the parasympathetic system in fear and anxiety, especially stress response theory framing the neurobiological context alongside an intervention that can help the two become unfused.

For example, someone who suffers from GAD may not be overly averse to the idea of any particular scenario occurring, but worries excessively that numerous bad things are more likely to occur to them than other people, contributing to their constant worrying and elevated anxiety levels. Someone who is frightened of dogs - a strong fear - would be averse to the idea of a dog attacking them. Lesser fears can exist at the same/similar time as having the main strong fear; anxiety is a lower level of anxiety. Furthermore, the context of experiences can shape them and whether they are perceived as fearful or anxiety-provoking.

In conclusion, fear and anxiety are both fairly normal feelings that are experienced by everyone at some point in their lives. While these two feelings seem somewhat interchangeable, or at the very least similar, upon closer inspection it becomes more obvious that the two are quite distinct from one another. If Whitney's explanations are to be agreed with, fear is both triggered and alleviated by very different factors than anxiety. Because of these differences, an individual may struggle with one emotion, while feeling very little in relation to the other.

In some cases, an evolutionary perspective can help elucidate why people experience fear or anxiety. A cognitive perspective can also provide a coherent explanation for both types of experiences people may have related to fear. With a better understanding of the brain's structure and functions, fear will be seen to have a deeper meaning. A human being's awareness of, or rational reflection in the face of, threat or danger manifests as an emotion. A dual process of automatic and controlled processing begins in the brain once emotional awareness sets in. In order to provide appropriate instructions for self-protection or problem-solving, the brain performs coordinated bulk motor output and perceptual awareness. So, pauses in such controlled processing give the mind time to engage with the threat and decide what to do about it.

Fear and anxiety are normal and helpful reactions in certain situations, but they are not interchangeable terms. Fear is often an emotional response to a clear and present danger, whereas anxiety is more often characterized by an anticipation of a potential future threat. Both fear and anxiety activate the body's "fight or flight" response, even though the stimulus and timeline of the threat differ. The conditions of phobia, panic disorder, and generalized anxiety disorder are all related to an unhealthy form of fear or anxiety.

8.2. Future Directions in Research

Research on anxiety, fear, and personality disorders remains an area ripe for continued exploration. Furthermore, while there is a tendency to focus on the negative consequences of states of fear or anxiety, it may also be beneficial to ascertain the role of these states in human development. For example, argue that "we need people who thrive on anxiety because we all genuinely like a bright future" (p. 1317), and such a person "...they outline ...maintain the highest quality and productiveness of the company" (p. 1317). The role necessity of anxiety appears to be more prominent in people in positions of power who are managing other people. As a result, "[a] normal distribution of anxiety as you move up the model of hierarchy in organizations is to be expected.

We came to the conclusion of this essay with the understanding that there are many aspects still to be discovered related to the nature of fear and anxiety, particularly within the etiology and treatment of anxiety-related disorders. This is especially true when considering the evolution of techniques designed to explore the neural systems underpinning these experiences, which are only now providing useful empirical data. The role of the different amygdala nuclei is still a topic of debate. It is clear that these various nuclei are involved in the different processes giving rise to fear or anxiety. With new neuroimaging techniques and the advent of nonhuman primate models of fear conditioning, new research directions are possible. This is an area of development which could also provide useful information about the etiology of disorders of fear and anxiety.

Understanding the Distinction Between Fear and Anxiety

1. Introduction to Fear and Anxiety

Fear has both an immediate and an expected future counterpart. The immediate one is typically distinguished as "fear," the future one as "fear," but sometimes as "fear of" or "anticipated fear." Correspondingly, anxiety typically accompanies both current, immediate behaviors and detectable signals such as restlessness, scanning, thermal-regulatory changes (like perspiration or panting), and activation of the rapid-autonomic-fear-system, as well as with an understandable and symmetrical future expectancy or anticipation of danger. In general, "fear" and "anxiety" occur in response to potential threats to survival and reproduction. Any given instance of fear or anxiety will have a minimal degree of two different types of information: one will be about the emotion itself (e.g., that the individual feels anxious or fearful), and the other will typically afford some awareness of what the threat is. "Threat" in the broadest sense includes anything that can deprive an individual of life, in a simple, direct, and immediate sense.

Introduction Fear and anxiety are both emotions, i.e., they are accompanied by specific, conscious "feelings." The terms are often used interchangeably, but in fact, they have very different meanings. The behavior that is called "fear" is almost always focused on some danger to the individual who feels it, while the behavior stereotypically called "anxiety" typically involves a diffuse attention to everything in the individual's environment, as if danger could be threatening from any direction, even though there is nothing specific to focus on as the source of the threat.

2. Historical Perspectives on Fear and Anxiety

For centuries, people have been attempting to understand our wide range of human emotional experiences. While many theories have tried to capture these complexities, perhaps two emotions that have stirred our imaginations more than any others are fear and anxiety. Already in the anxiety literature, there is a very ancient and global distinction of long standing between fear and 'dread'. She suggests that the anxiety of continents hence has been around a long time. There are numerous similarly ancient and nonwesternly distinctions between these two experiences. For example, the distinction between American Indian tribe members is also already present in Iroquois accounts of "the great beast of personal fear, that other fear we call anxiety" noted in 1696 by Dekanawida and Hiawatha but also marked in Algonquin oral culture of the Neutrals and the Huron and by Ongwehonwe people as "this greeting of fear" in the 1200s. Gradually the name-dread, carried from the Mohegans to the Pequots in the 1600s, changed with settlers into the meaning-"the evil eye"-at the same time it entered all the histories of the New England with a different name, black dagon.

Fear is a necessary, nonpathological defensive response to a real, present threat. It is the sudden and intense expression of panic, bloody fear, that purchases time for a more reflective action to be taken. Anxiety is a connected emotion that can be both adaptive and dysfunctional, but it is tied to a future threat that is either unknown, diffuse or of uncertain timing. It is a state in which the threat is in the process of being anticipated.

3. Neurobiological Basis of Fear and Anxiety

The emotional and physiological expressions of anxiety take several forms that include autonomic and hormonal changes, such as increased heart rate, salivation, perspiration, pupil dilation, tensed muscles, and slowing of digestion. Anxiety also involves an increased startle reaction, constant scanning of the environment (vigilance), and further hyperactivity of the HPA axis, especially during the pre-novelty period (i.e. approach to the start of a potentially feared activity). The central nuclei of the amygdala are necessary for an association between a threatening or unpleasant stimulus (a noxious unconditioned stimulus or an aversive conditioned stimulus) and the fear elicited. The basolateral nuclei of the amygdala contain an internal model of the world built up through complex interaction with the associative cortices, and which is manipulated through the value systems of the individual. Separable, though interconnected, neural circuits and neurotransmitter systems also underlie the control of fear and anxiety. In general, the mechanisms of the "fear control system" are under greater cognitive regulation than those of the "anxiety/behavioral inhibition system."

The experience of anxiety is both complex and multifaceted and involves several components, including elements of negative affect, behavioral inhibition, and a hypervigilant anticipation of future disaster. Since many elements behaviorally and phenomenologically associated with anxiety are also part of one's behavioral repertoire in the face of fear, some have suggested that fear and anxiety are one and the same, differing only in terms of the imponderables of eliciting events or their threshold for elicitation. While the exact nature of the relationship between fear and anxiety awaits further research, evidence suggests that anxiety, as well as fear, is formed from subcortically mediated, danger-based responses that are adapted to facing dangerous environments.

4. Psychological Theories of Fear and Anxiety

It is most certainly true that the distinction between fear and anxiety is a pivotal theoretical and clinical issue, particularly in domains where development is examined. Although the syntagmatic opposition has a history in philosophical theories of affect, modern theorizing surrounding differences between these two has taken shape predominantly in terms of attitude or approach on one hand, or as conceptual gradience, on the other. Althusser, for example, claims that fear is the experience of a danger present but may possibly be determined and controlled. By contrast, anxiety, in his sense, is merely the encounter of an absence or "a hole." In apprehending such, the fearful subject is "certain to know nothing about the terror which possesses him or the reason which governs it." Insofar as we take a critical view of polemical differences, Althusser begins to provide an example of a reader who confuses the two opposite sides of the distinction.

Some regard Freud as a figure who gave voice to humanity's darkest fears and anxieties. However, there is a particular kind of suffering we can experience that Freud, indeed, prefers to leave to others to look into; as Green (1996) argues, Freud always kept a certain distance from anxiety proper. One may even go as far as wonder if anxiety resists psychoanalytic analysis altogether seeing as Freud's sense of this emotion has subsequently been colored by the proliferation of psychoanalytic interpretations, most notably in the way selected analysts have accompanied the clinical work and writings of Heidegger (e.g., Pollock). When encountering such self-preserving distances that some (assumingly Freud too) may wish to maintain in relation to the temporality and modality of anxiety, we are faced with questions that cut across several interrelated domains that the philosopher and psychoanalyst must confront in their respective inquiries into both temporality and the experiential world.

5. Emotional and Physiological Responses to Fear and Anxiety

Physiological responses. When danger is sensed, the body undergoes a "fight-or-flight response." This response generally occurs in reaction to a large real or imagined incursion that exceeds the resources of a person, thereby necessitating a response of immediate defense or escape. Characteristic of the moment of fear is the activation of the adrenal medulla, resulting in the release of adrenaline (sparking an increase in heart rate), and the activation of the hypothalamus, resulting in the release of cortisol from the adrenal cortex. On the other hand, anxiety is elicited by a non-real or anticipated future or imagined threat and does not contain the same fight-or-flight reaction. In this instance, a mild to moderate response is initiated.

Emotional responses. The responses set off by fear and anxiety are comprised of both emotional and physiological reactions. These complex responses encompass cognitions, behaviors, autonomic reactions, and endocrine secretion. It is common to speak of "feeling anxiety," but in reality this phrase encompasses three different ways of experiencing anxiety. According to Hopp, anxiety refers to "(a) an emotional state that arises from the negative appraisal of perceived external threat; (b) an aversive emotional state that arises from focusing attention on interoceptive or somatic cues (e.g., increased heart rate) or from uncertainty about the existence of a pathological somatic state; or (c) an aversive emotional state associated with anxious cognition (e.g., worry) in the absence of immediate external threat that is interoceptive-focused, concerned with uncertainty, or concerned with a variety of bad things that might happen in the future."

6. Cognitive Processes in Fear and Anxiety

Attention and the Cognitive Availability of Threat Information. The influence of attention on the perception of fear and anxiety has been enriched. Different from anxiety, attention shifting is disrupted in pathological fear, especially in the presence of unpredictable threatening events. In addition, there are reports indicating that individuals with pathological fear are more prone to overload of working memory. Recent research described that non-clinical worry and generalized anxiety disorders generate Fear-Threat Equivalent (ant) Stimuli. The threats and their ambiguity in worry, similar to pathological fear, seem to roughly share the same cognitive processor with the same dysfunctionality. However, imagination is another powerful tool of cognitive appraisal that is used to release the perceived threat. When used as an adaptive tool, imagination tries to see and act upon a number of future possibilities in gaining control of it. Cognitive inflexibility contrarily occurs in real sudden feared threat in habituated neurological responses (fear) resulting in sudden irrelevant cognitive modifications (confabulation), often seen in NAc (nucleus accumbens) tumor patients.

Cognitive Processes in Fear and Anxiety. How individuals think when they are in fear and anxiety is one of the main processes that distinguish fear and anxiety. Different from fear where the threat is present, anxiety is a condition where it is seen as an uncertainty threat. Information that is processed in anxious people (not yet threatened) is often in the domain of danger or self-minimizing catastrophic outcome. They have the tendency to see a range of events as a possible negative outcome, to underestimate their control over these outcomes, to produce negative images in their minds, and to delay seeking a solution. Anxious people seem to work harder to suppress a negative image or thought from memory than do non-anxious individuals. The main problem of anxiety is when the individual does not release the anxious state and keeps ruminating around the possibility of the occurrence threat. Normally, fear and anxiety are involved with multiple cognitive biases that construe and enhance the appraisals of threat and danger. Cognitive revaluation (CR), also, serves as a mitigating strategy for the cognitive process that is not present in the fear response due to cognitive inflexibility from the amygdala. Therefore, people in anxiety (future-oriented) are trying to discover a way to release the threat from their cognitive appraisal. It could be known in the form of checking behaviors, avoidance behavior, or reassuring behavior. Cognitive inflexibility when facing a sudden threat occurs in fear (present and real threat) and is often processed confabulatorily. Cognitive biases in fear also directly enhance attentional shift to possible negative events and quickly gain initiated by subcortical amygdala.

7. Developmental Aspects of Fear and Anxiety

Let us first turn to fear. This emotion is considered to be a human universal potentially observable across the world. While certain phobias tend to appear at particular periods of life, numerous fears can be found at most or many periods of life. Those typical of young children include hospitals, health and death, ghosts, as well as the dark or ghosts and the supernatural. On average, what changes in the average number of fears between infancy and childhood is the nature of the like and the common, i.e., both fears and favorite preferences tend to concern the environment. In contrast, fears common to teenagers are mostly social. The quality of children's fears and phobias tends to change with age. In addition, the sensations and behaviors elicited by the fear which concern children involve more behaviors and physical symptoms than serving children. The greatest number of physical and behavioral changes linked to fear is hyperventilation. In adolescence, fears appear to be much less frequent than in preceding ages. What resemble 'fears' show fear, anger, and being worried.

Human development theories emphasize the roots of human emotion, mentioning its various early signs as an instinct, an inherited response. This chapter will show, however, that this focus is more than anything else on fear - on early signs of fear's development. Indeed, distinct types of fear develop and are displayed at different times of life. Most importantly, feelings about fear change with age. From an early age, people claim not to be afraid of potential objects of fear that they considered to be threatening in the past. How can this assertion be understood?

8. Cultural and Social Influences on Fear and Anxiety

Patel makes a distinction between some societies, which understand the greatest part of the phenomena and emotions which may possibly generate one of the two compensatory processes (punishment and trial-procedure) in terms of fear controls and, finally, use them to put some kind of sanctions, and the "modern" societies. These latter ones, beginning from the nineteenth century value all of the negatives only in terms of anxiety, in the next sense of worrying. Before the nineteenth century, anxiety and fear were not well distinguished even in Western societies. In the classical world the term anxiety simply means celibacy, while the last name Anxur means Jupiter, who gave patients a dream making them well within his sanctuary. In the Western world anxiety is considered by Pattison not to have a long past: its social ascension only succeeds its medical one. He explains it due to the idea one had around 1750 of the human mind, which represents the first organic conception of man.

Fear is more likely to be associated with physical harm, with the anticipation of abrupt dangers, while anxiety is more socio-emotional, linked to the anticipation of future troubles in the context of the lack of information (its cognitive basis). The role of the socio-cultural environment in the distinction between fear and anxiety is much more complex. It does not seem that there exist cultures dominated by one of the two emotions; rather some societies are dominated by fear (as most of the traditional societies), while in others the experience and expression of anxiety is quite spread (as in modern Western ones). Among tribes that have been studied there is a strong link between the personality of the individual who fears (in large societies) and the objects of fear. However, for us, it is interesting to examine the transcultural aspects of the distinction, which make it possible to substantiate the emotional attitudes specific to either fear or anxiety.

9. Clinical Manifestations of Fear and Anxiety Disorders

The degree to which anxiety is disproportionate may be either normal or pathological. Anxiety is a symptom that can occur at any time in disorders such as major depression, mania, bipolar disorder, and schizophrenia. The most common form of psychological disorder among the general population is anxiety disorder. In the case of anxiety, the ability to accurately appraise dangerous situations is compromised; for fear to be adaptive, it must coincide with the occurrence of a real threat. ACCT also highlights the factors that account for selective disturbance of this ability. Natural Selection Theory allows us to isolate the universal features of all fears and invert fears such that they would support the optimal realization of scared feelings and the beliefs and drives that index them. Scared feelings are normatively accompanied by corresponding beliefs and drives. It is similar to hope, which is a belief accompanied by a drive to seek and an anticipation of favorable outcomes. On the other hand, medically unjustified fears or misguided fears are considered abnormal. Only from this approach can we explain the pseudoneurotic distress and depressive despair that patients with misdirected fears demonstrate. The diagnosis of fear-borne illness must confirm that the distressing fear violates the patient's beliefs, goals, or other earlier adaptive concerns, not some recent internal forces or situation that will pass with time; this is why the fear causes excessive distress. If measure of distress is shown (subjectively, by verbal communication, facial expression, various psychophysiological measures, etc.), appropriate plans of action can be made.

Nature to provide a focused discussion related to clinical perspective. Both fear and anxiety disorders come with excessive difficulties in thinking, controlling, and otherwise managing fear or anxiety. Irrational fears cause irrational responses and urges, while depression may also be present. The response of both situationally predisposed and situationally predisposed fears can be characterized by selective processing of threatening information. Clinical anxiety, according to DSM-5, can be comprehensively divided into five categories: social anxiety disorder, panic disorder, generalized anxiety disorder, agoraphobia, and specific phobias. Social anxiety disorder presents with a constant fear that one might be negatively evaluated in social situations. Chronic fear describes an unrealistic and excessive form of emotions. A clinical diagnosis is diagnosed if symptoms occur for six months, cause emotional distress, interfere with daily functioning, and are not attributable to another psychological condition. Acute anxiety regarding loved ones or social situations is a universal experience for everyone. However, the independence which is diagnosed clinically is based on the existence of urge, duration, and interference with daily functioning.

10. Assessment and Diagnosis of Fear and Anxiety Disorders

If a dichotomous diagnosis can be made, many assessment tools for fear and anxiety can be patented as diagnostic tests. In this connection, many questionnaires, rating scales, and structured and semi-structured interviews have been described in the chapter so that the readers can make an independent choice of the test according to the clinical and research situation. Like other mental disorders, the diagnosis of anxiety can also be made on the basis of careful history, mental status examination, and physical and laboratory examination. However, many authors have developed structured and semi-structured interviews and questionnaires for the diagnosis of anxiety disorders. Chapter 4, therefore, focuses on various rating scales, questionnaires, structured interviews, semi-structured interviews, and physical and laboratory examinations. Chapter 5 further describes the clinical examination of anxiety disorders based on DSM-III, DSM-III-R, DSM-IV, and ICD-10 classification. Assessment of fear and anxiety should be an integral part of the clinical management of all mental disorders. In Section B, the chapter lists the differential diagnostic states of fear and anxiety that should be kept in mind.

As Kar et al. have rightly said, there has been a remarkable shift in the focus of research from syndromic diagnoses (normal sadness, normal fear, and psychotic fear) to nosologic diagnoses (fear symptom syndromes, fear disorders) (p. 159). In our perception, along with focusing on this nosologic diagnosis, it is pertinent both theoretically and practically to be able to make a distinction between the intense pathological fear (fear disorder) and anxiety (anxiety disorder), as it has a bearing not only on the treatment and longitudinal outcome of the patient but also on clinical and basic neuroscience research and application of the research findings in clinical practice. We have discussed the clinical and therapeutic implications in detail in Chapter 12 (Assessment and Differential Diagnosis of Intense Pathological Fear and Anxiety).

10. Assessment and Diagnosis of Fear and Anxiety Disorders

From the book: Multiple Faces of Fear: The Expert Guide to Neuroses

11. Treatment Approaches for Fear and Anxiety Disorders

Treatment approaches for fear and anxiety disorders. Effective mental healthcare for individuals living with fear and anxiety symptoms make use of a variety of modalities and models. There are a number of evidence-based treatments that employ different scientific theories and therapeutic techniques with the aim of reducing and controlling fear, anxiety, and other mental health symptoms and promoting well-being. On the one hand, cognitive-behavioral therapy can include psychoeducation about mental health challenges, cognitive restructuring to challenge negative automatic thoughts, behavioral activation to increase rewarding activities, and/or behavioral exposure to reduce avoidance and decrease only when combined with cognitive restructuring. Pharmacologic therapies may be used differently in the treatment of fear and anxiety symptoms. For post-traumatic stress disorder, sertraline and paroxetine are the first-line treatments, while for social anxiety disorder, fluoxetine and paroxetine have shown efficacy. Evidence demonstrates that a combination of pharmacologic therapy, specifically some selective serotonin reuptake inhibitors, and cognitive-behavioral exposure therapy provide the most effective treatment for people with obsessive-compulsive disorder. Noninvasive brain stimulation methods can also be used alongside counseling for specific clinical populations, as well as for others and in clinical trials. Moreover, at an exploratory level, mobile health and therapies (e.g., tailored online therapy) can also be used to complement other clinical interventions.

Fear and anxiety: Overlapping processes. Fear and anxiety processing often intersect; one can arise from another. In the first, it is argued that fear is an ingrained environmental response to a real, present, or imminent physical or emotional threat, while anxiety is a future-oriented perspective on threat involving the sense of control. Another model of the fear-anxiety relationship is based on avoidance or escape responses, where fear comprises an immediate physiological response to environmental threat or danger, enabling an individual to defend themselves or flee. In contrast to fear, anxiety is described as indefinite apprehension or tension about future events, specifically those that may result in harm or a stressful situation.

12. Prevention and Coping Strategies for Fear and Anxiety

• Resilience Development: Children should be given coping strategies that build up resilience and encourage growth. Bordow and Porch encourage educators to teach children "resiliency" skills. A resilient child will approach life with hope and confidence rather than fear. For young children, physical activity should be used to burn off some of the stress. Baseball games, skateboarding clinics or bike safety rodeos will help children "think forward." This kind of thinking will help reduce the chances of clinical anxiety and fears from developing. • Coping Mechanisms: Teaching children coping methods can help them manage anxiety and stress. Young children can draw a picture of their family or write their fears down on a piece of paper and stomp it or tear it up. Relaxation methods such as deep breathing, visual imagery or muscle relaxation can also help children deal with their fears. Provide young people with skills for constructive action by listening attentively, providing emotional support, encouraging peer support and redirecting children's energy toward participation in or contributions toward constructive activities.

Practitioners should consider several coping strategies and resilience-building techniques by which individuals and communities may insulate themselves to effectively manage and recover from acute events such as terrorism, or in coping with chronic unpredictable events such as warfare. These strategies are adaptable to broader community strategies. Thus, it is sought to foster plans based upon local needs, potential disruption, individual characteristics and coping strategies reflecting local culture and capacity.

13. Fear and Anxiety in Specific Populations

Fear and anxiety are prevalent, though distinct, diseases among children. Specific to post-traumatic stress disorders, including fear and anxiety, a notable amount of research has focused on understanding the basic roles fear plays in the development of anxiety disorders among children. Assessed following the September 11, 2001, events, Preiss et al. found a strong relationship between race and levels of severe fear in children; a possible outcome of racial profiling and discrimination. The study was conducted in a low-income, largely minority school district in the Midwest. This suggests that living in an already precarious environment exacerbates the fear response in a devastating way.

Fear and anxiety are diseases that present in unique ways depending on the patient's age, gender, and many other demographic variables. Among adults, females are twice as likely to experience anxiety than males, and children exhibit a similar disparity. Furthermore, symptoms of anxiety disorders were often experienced differently between the sexes than those of the other sex. Also, among the adult population, though somewhat predictive of anxiety symptoms, several factors such as race, education, marital status, and job class were significant influences on fear and its underlying causes. As a result, in treating differences in anxiety symptomology, many factors must be taken into account, including gender, age, sexuality, race, and many others, in order to best understand the etiology of fear and anxiety and the unique approach needed with specific patients.

14. Fear and Anxiety in the Workplace

In addition, cultures or the reverse (An)surveillance can replicate the psychological features of anxiety that presumes that one's self is always potentially on display without the individual being capable of identifying from whence or from whom the possible surveillance emanates. These psychological conditions speak to more immediate occupational concerns and the anxieties that develop in the face of imposed occupational stress from above. At universities, in the 1980s, a number of scholars faced anxieties and depression as a result of imposed research regimes. In the workplace, fear and anxiety can be fomented through poor work relations, with crafting each person into an individualization of organizing rights and wrongs.

While, from the psychological perspective, fear and anxiety are characterized by the anticipation of, or response to, a real or imagined threat or event, they are often illustrated distinctively through accounts that relate to some of the significant workplace experiences. Gilbert discusses the role that a culture of blame and performance management heightens fears of exposure, actual or not, and his 'fear management continuum' can be illustrated in Cameron et al's work, following the managerialist and functionalist perspective that promotes organizational well-being. Cameron et al conceptualize employees with good mental ill-being 'tapped on the shoulder' by visible distress and anxiety where they are insufficiently equipped to function in promised high-performing roles. They suggest a workplace where training and development provide individuals with the 'necessary tools' to perform to such standards, building a 'thicker' resilience that values new competencies to sharpen up workers' emotional and social abilities, promoting a more generic psychological well-being that furthers domination. As a result, a fear of being exposed in terms of occupationally unacceptable attributes and subsequent anxiety reflects a dynamic shaped by performance expectations and skills fitting into an economically dominated landscape marked by alienation.

15. Fear and Anxiety in Educational Settings

Research has shown that children will perform tasks and garner recommendations based on an adult's contributed anxiety level. The overwhelming majority of research on teacher effects has focused on academic achievement. In recent years, schools have started to focus on student developmental outcomes such as socio-emotional and noncognitive factors, experiencing increased interest from policymakers, with broad implications for the education and health fields. Increased attention is given to the relationship between noncognitive skills, conditions in the classroom that foster such skills, and children's long-term educational and economic outcomes. Key to this meta-analysis is fear that the focus has expanded to promote positive socio-emotional attributes associated with academic achievement.

Fear and anxiety can be prevalent in educational environments. While few studies have focused on two of the most common emotions experienced by children in educational settings, it is evident that anxiety permeates almost every aspect of the child's life and is experienced by the child as perpetually near. Other research has found that a variety of stressors, from interpersonal relationships with teachers, homework, poverty, and racial discrimination, contribute to children's fear and anxiety. Other childhood factors associated with anxiety include academic pressures and a negative school climate characterized by problematic teacher-student relationships and lack of student support from teachers and schools. Recent sports research highlighting developmental experiences for Black teenagers living in stigmatized urban environments also emphasizes the level of anxiety associated with institutional fear in relationships with prejudiced police officers affiliated with urban public schools, experiences that the authors call "learning fear." This author's research emphasizes the use of educational curricula that promote safe and supportive learning environments.

16. Fear and Anxiety in the Media and Entertainment Industry

The public is continuing to have an evident interest in terrorism and political violence (and also in health threats) where media plays a significant role. Indeed, millions of people appreciate – that is to say, give their "appreciation" (in the original sense of "being worthy of our thanks") – the finest media that expose parts of the globe we have never even heard of pack specific emotional effects between their commercials. The more exotic and "unfamiliar" a location is shown in the news coverage, the more "fear" this coverage creates. All known studies have shown that viewers give preference to the causes and consequences of traumatic fears and anxieties rather than the predictable ones such as the disintegration of a virtual "European Society".

Moving away from philosophy and religion, fear and anxiety are highly represented in media and entertainment, where artists translate different feelings about themselves, their creatures, and the audience. So, actually, media and professionals who work in the entertainment industry and mass media "have made a killing through what you pay to watch." Producers of entertainment and news professionals manage fear and anxiety openings as spaces for commercial exploitation. At the same time, fear and anxiety in the media can be aimed at learning, establishing preventive measures not only for personal security but also to protect people with whom we lead a life in common. That is why, increasing fears and anxieties is not necessarily a bad thing. In fact, the increase of security and preventive mechanisms is based on the creation of fears and anxieties. Different fears and anxieties are created in order to adopt security and preventive measures and some fears and some anxieties are expressed to create consent against risking in. But caring for ourselves at all times is also a "cure" for collective living; in other words, the more secure we are, the more secure those with whom we live are.

17. Fear and Anxiety in Literature and Art

In visual arts, traditional focal figures of fear are ghostly apparitions, demonic elements, or ugly misshapen to human nature deformed bodies. Less direct into the public's unconscious, anxiety induces the very specific sense of paradox and withdraw from either/or thinking, proposing a subtle class of psycho-poetic conceptual artworks, very conscious of the linguistic trap of the double bind. The anti-human artworks provoke a sort of existential-interpretivist paradox of abandoning their expression. It seems obvious that when addressing issues of fear and anxiety, these affective states are treated as presenting the dark side of any given artistic or literary narrative. Literary violence and cinema, as its most brightly colored and noisiest branch, through copy-some landscapes of violence, thus offers an indirect portal to the paranoid scenarios of fear and the future prefaced throughout the universe of creative endeavor.

Since ancient times, fear and anxiety have been themes that have seen countless representations in all kinds of artistic expression, literature, art, and performances. Some have even claimed that fear and anxiety are themes that can be found at the core of any artistic expression, as the moment of momentum that sustains the narrative movement. With regard to the thematic representation of fear and anxiety in art, there has been a two-fold interpretation. The main intention of modernists was to dismember and question the innermost logic of fear and anxiety. Even if artists and writers could not expect to replace philosophical expertise, they have undoubtedly become convincing propagandists and instinctual leaders of an altered form of fearful and anxious experience.

18. Fear and Anxiety in Philosophy

What is the nature of fear and anxiety? To what kinds of things can fear and anxiety be directed? What defines them? Are they feelings, emotions, passions or affects? How different are they from ordinary emotions like anger, sadness, joy, compassion? What is common between the two and what does distinguish them from other or each other?

Similarly to fear, in this case anxiety was also touched by distinctive debates in philosophy, like the existential one, where the problem was to define anxiety as "fear of nothing", where "nothing" depicts a special kind of object (or non-object), i.e. not an ordinary fear-object. Therefore, we do have more or less acknowledged distinctions attributable to the thinkers who approached this issue in philosophy, even though we still lack a wide reaching critical discussion to them. But, more importantly, we do not have an appraisal neither about what the various distinguishings should/could at the end concern, be around and deal.

Philosophy has always been intrigued by the phenomenon of fear. Ranging from existential considerations to ethical and metaphysical issues about reasons for action, way of behaving in the face of objects and attitudes to favour, distinct aspects have been analysed in the intricate set of aspects around fear. It is only recently that some space has also been given to anxiety as a phenomenon distinguishable from fear and worry. However, this debate is quite marginal and does not have the same depth as anxiety.

19. Fear and Anxiety in Religion and Spirituality

Theological and philosophical reflections on fear and anxiety include analyses of their relationships to faith, hope, charity, and despair, as well as historical attempts to integrate fear and anxiety into the ascetical practices and mystical attunements of particular religious and spiritual traditions. In addition, these mediations also reflect on the eschatological context within which fears may be sublimated in religious belief and devotional practices; new "affects" and attitudes could be generated that diminish or completely remove fears or anxiety. Spiritual practices and religious narratives that engage and recode fear and anxiety offer fresh insights, then, into the complex relationships between spiritual and affective dynamics.

Fear and anxiety are often thought to be part of the human experience and of interest to individual personality, mood, and motivation. This does not mean that there is no place to think about an emotion of the emotions or to think about fear and anxiety in more collective registers. For example, common to many definitions is the idea that an emotion is a mental phenomenon focused on the actual or likely dangers and troubles of the subject and that it inspires a range of responses to these threats or challenges. An emotional life extends over time and thus includes a range of moods, concerns, and dispositions that we associate with the appraisal of the personal, social, and material worlds. Detailing the relationship and distinction between emotion and mood requires more consideration of the phenomenological aspects of discrete affective states and activities; much philosophical and theological, as well as psychotherapeutic writing, moves rather easily among fear, anxiety, and dread without too much concern as to where one ends and the other begins.

20. Fear and Anxiety in Politics and Society

It is thought that fear and anxiety guide valuable policies such as environmental, health or social policies. Proponents of the hypothesis of the emotion compossibility are not only concerned with the nature of public policies that may respond to collective emotions, but also with a more basic question: are we ever right to respond to afflictive or negative emotions in the public domain? It is central to critically inquire into the normative dimensions of the public's reactions to feelings of fear and anxiety. Such considerations can be linked to social policy, insofar as social policy is concerned with the ways in which feelings of fear or anxiety may harm individuals and groups in our society. An additional question arises with regard to the sociopolitical considerations of the compossibility hypothesis, and it is important to address whether we ever should cultivate responsive public policies.

Recently, many integrated accounts of fear and anxiety have stressed the intersection of these emotions with political and societal discourses. Fear and anxiety, it seems, have important societal implications that are relevant for policy considerations. In liberal conceptions of politics, an agent's feelings, emotions or experiences are not external to the policy process, but rather have sociopolitical dimensions. Moreover, emotions are also intentional experiences that are essentially involved in the relational aspect of our being in the world. Not only do anxiety or fear have societal implications, engendering a vast amount of literature on risk society, they may also involve political rhetoric. One might view hesitations with regard to policy proposals that affect or exploit feelings of fear or anxiety as ethical scruple about the use of political rhetoric.

21. Fear and Anxiety in Environmental Contexts

To dig beneath the notion of existential integration, we continue to operate using some of Max Scheler's basic psychological premises from nearly a century ago. First, persons, for Scheler, are characterized by a tendency to visualize our fundamental connection to other beings and "values" in either of two basic ways. First, we often visualize our "formal" or intrinsic similarities and differences with a variety of other beings, including other humans. Second, we are also usually influenced by how others treat us and how we treat them, focusing on the "experiential" or instrumental qualitatively environmental aspects of our relationships, especially our interpersonal ones. Scheler's third and final psychological devotion to our environmental heritage secured individuals in their place in the cosmos.

In other words, these items that are most the source of fear and anxiety terminate in a concept or series of contents that largely alter the categories that we humans use in our science and the way of living towards the world. In particular, the quantum nature of life changes our views of causality and introduces purpose, the nuclear nature of life alters, as in Aeschylus, our views of the relationship between technical skill and our own fate. Khimotronomondo, that about which all of us must be the most concerned, involves an ecologically constrained understanding of economics, politics, and science.

The items of greatest environmental concern at the moment, those that are most anguishing to great numbers of beings and that are the source, as we feel it, of much of the frantic activity preferred by many people (which we label anxiety), are climate change, nuclear weapons and nuclear plants, biological invasion, waters that carry poisons, animals that stave off infection, and quantum mechanics. These items contain two main sub-categories. Both the primal nature of some items, the scope of others, and the extent of the damage wrought in all cases by selfishness and fear, is intensely ecological.

First, we turn to some of the ways in which people use the terms "fear" and "anxiety." Abstracting from any psychological or biological specificity, fear is most often used to indicate a present (real, potential, or imagined) harm, while anxiety is used to indicate a threat that is far off and as unavoidable as it is anticipated. People sometimes disagree about where to draw the line, on either time or the reality/potentiality distinctions. While there are many possible cues for varying the use of these words, we think that attending to the role of other beings and things in evoking these states is instructive. To some extent, a common way to discuss a distinction between fear and anxiety is through emphasizing the role and scope of the information available to the person experiencing such states, including her degree of initial certainty about the harmfulness of the situation. We are almost always interested in the environmental influences and effects. There are significant differences in the ways in which environments affect fear and anxiety. This is partly the extent to which the environment requires at its adaptation organs, or some complicated aspect of the mind, though it is also influenced by the meanings and social attributes of different environments. All of that said, humans have always recognized that stressors in the environment can be proximally perceived, triggering "fear" and that our home environment influences the minutiae of our moods, including feelings of "anxious dread."

22. Fear and Anxiety in the Digital Age

Despite the unavoidable turns to affect in public discourse and the myriad of affect-related research fields (the always growing names of those who "study feeling"), and despite the not-so-innate biological ground of affect, fear and anxiety have emerged as frames of discontent that play off of darker diagnostics of extreme malaise, mental illness, and ensemble disorders of virtual hypochondria. Some owners of our emerging digital worlds have accordingly gestured toward, or considered to incorporate, the management of fear and anxiety as part of the menu of services such enterprises have to offer.

While digital affects have emboldened these conditions, there are additional threads in affect theory that require attention. There is the realm of speculative critique, where emotions have been situated as a resource to frame discussions of "intelligent" bodies or thinkers, or are posed as vestiges of a prior time "when biology still mattered." Fear and anxiety here support epistemological cleavages.

It is true in this digitally attuned environment that we are more or less positioned to encounter others as fundamentally emotional entities, either prone to emotional argument or as embodiments of affect-ridden discourses.

The histories of these psychological states and their cultural manifestations often relegated in affect theory to biological and neurological interpretations suggest that in the United States or some other similarly digitized societies, the scale and scope of people's experience of the world is now inflected by these conditions of the digital. The implications of this sensibility for experience similarly spill over into discussions about the categorization of what is deemed either real or at the mercy of neurological force, conditioned as impact or event.

In digital times, how we experience fear and anxiety has increasingly drawn the attention of scholars and popular culture. Digital technology, as we read echoes often in academic and public debates, purportedly changes the nature and affective tenor of these psychological states, which are then further understood to resonate across personal life, politics, and other social domains.

23. Future Directions in Fear and Anxiety Research

This chapter highlighted future areas for research based on exciting new results in fear and anxiety research. While some of the areas are emerging, for example, individuals are just beginning to realize the problems associated with the large gaps between the two main levels of analyses that constitute the divisions within Division 30: Biological. Indeed, it is likely that few members of Division 30 were even aware of these gaps at the time of this writing. Clearly, then, this review was not an attempt to microscopically spell out every direction that fear and anxiety research should be, or is likely to be, headed, but it was instead intended to be a provocative and lively overview of some of the most pressing and important issues that currently face the field.

Fear and anxiety research has made tremendous progress over the past half century, leading to a detailed understanding of the neural circuits, genes, molecules, and cells that control these complex states. This understanding has also contributed to a wave of new treatments for anxiety and related disorders. This article outlines the authors' views on some exciting new areas for future research. We focus on the development of technological tools that allow for the exquisite interrogation and manipulation of neurons, genes, and circuits. We also stress the increasing importance of studying anxiety along and across the lifespan, from development to extinction to relapse. Finally, we suggest that innovative therapies could arise from combining traditionally distinct levels of analysis and drawing on expertise from different disciplinary perspectives. In conclusion, the fast pace of technological and social change is placing pressure on our twenty-year-old systems of research and classification in ways that have never been greater. Emerging new research frontiers offer valuable opportunities to develop new biologically grounded approaches to both diagnosis and therapy.